OSCAR OCEAN AND THE BIG SMILE

JOSEPHINE N.C. GROENHART

ISBN: 1535485833
ISBN-13: 978-1535485838

DEDICATION

For the amazing children we see in our centre taking on new and exciting challenges. Enjoy your journey.

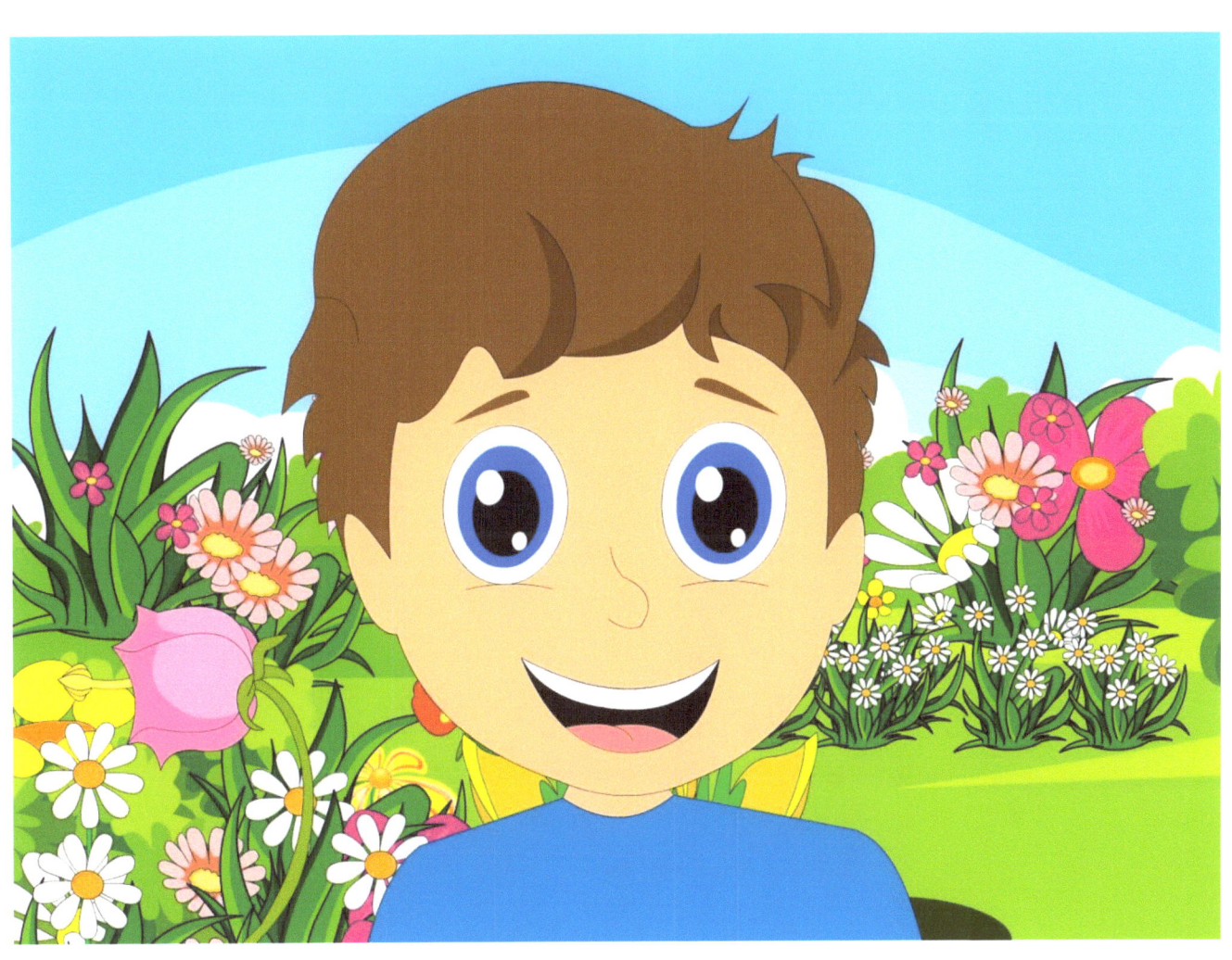

ACKNOWLEDGMENTS

With special thanks to Ambadi Kumar for her amazing illustrations, Ed for all your encouragement and Isaac, Oakley and all the children in our centre who have helped me put this together for you all.

THANK YOU

Oscar was sitting alone on the floor,

More Grumpy than we have ever seen before.

His new bike now thrown to one side

Stomping and shouting as his face he did hide

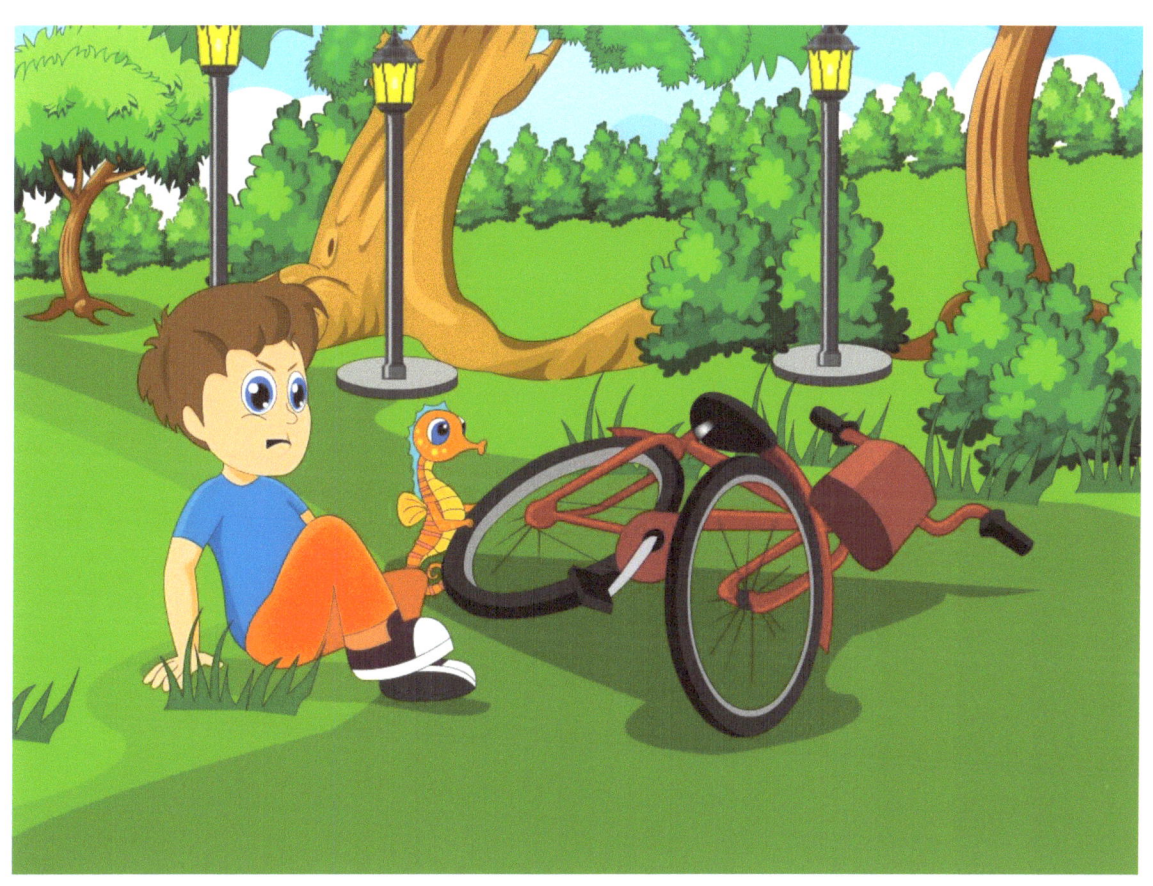

Of course now we wonder

As we look and ponder

What has occurred here with Oscar today?

Why has his bike been pushed away?

Sammy Seahorse said, "Oh Oscar you were doing so well,

But then by accident you swerved and fell.

Never mind though Oscar, it's really fine

And only to be expected at this time."

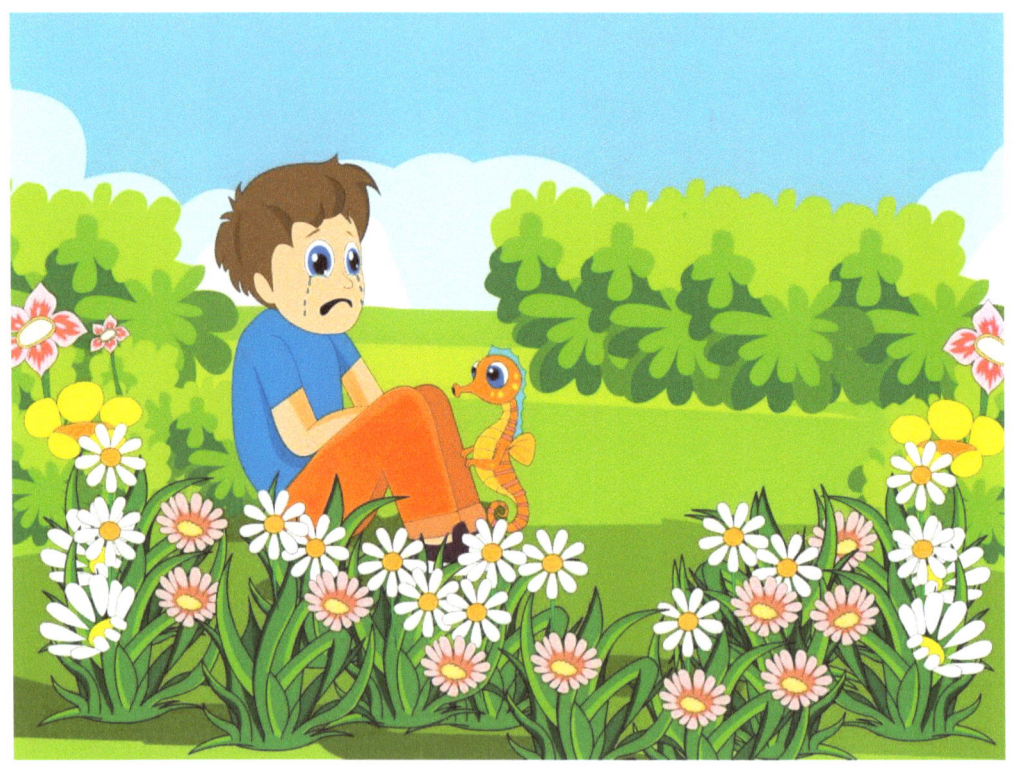

"But I just can't do it, Oscar grumbled,

I can't ride my bike and then I tumbled

It's not fair. It's no good. I can't ride."

Then shouting and screaming he stood and cried.

Standing close by, Sammy stopped still,

"Of course you can't ride and you never will!

Your mood is foul and your attitude rotten

Come on Oscar, PMA, have you forgotten?"

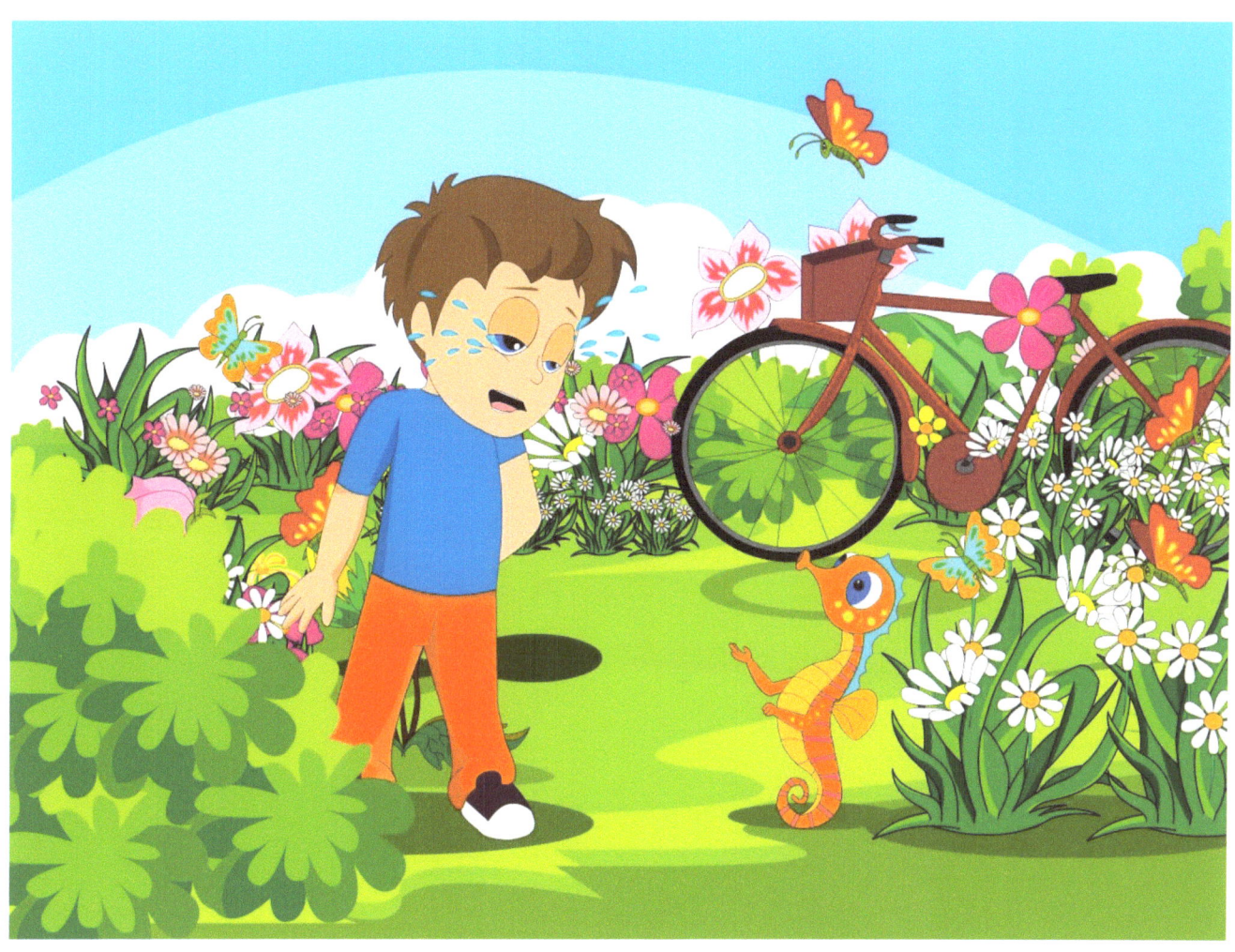

Puzzled Oscar raised his head

"PMA? What's PMA? He simply said

"Oh dear," said Sammy, "you're in a muddle

Let's find our friends. Quick at the double!"

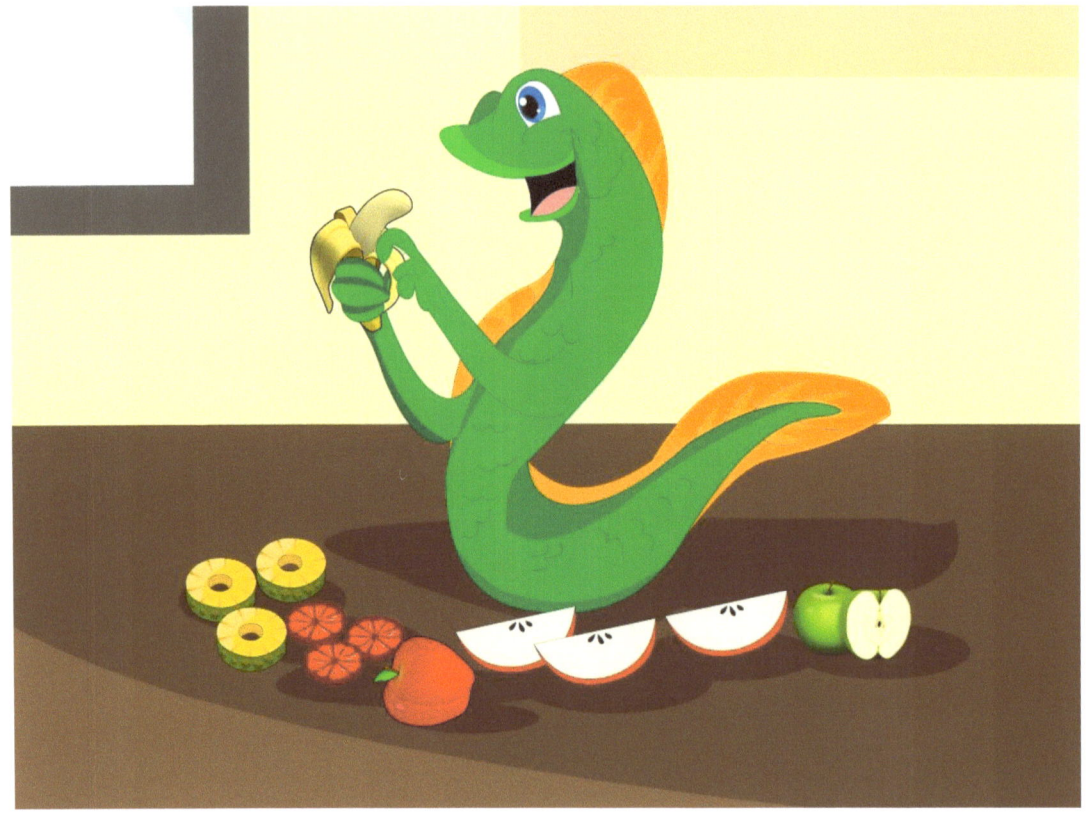

"Come on Emily eel, where are you?"

Shouted Sammy, "Oscar is in a bit of a stew."

Emily appeared from under a bush,

"Hello there Sammy, what's the rush?"

"Oscar has forgotten his PMA

It's gone; it's lost its fizzled away.

Emily we need the team to help explain

Why PMA is important for growth and gain."

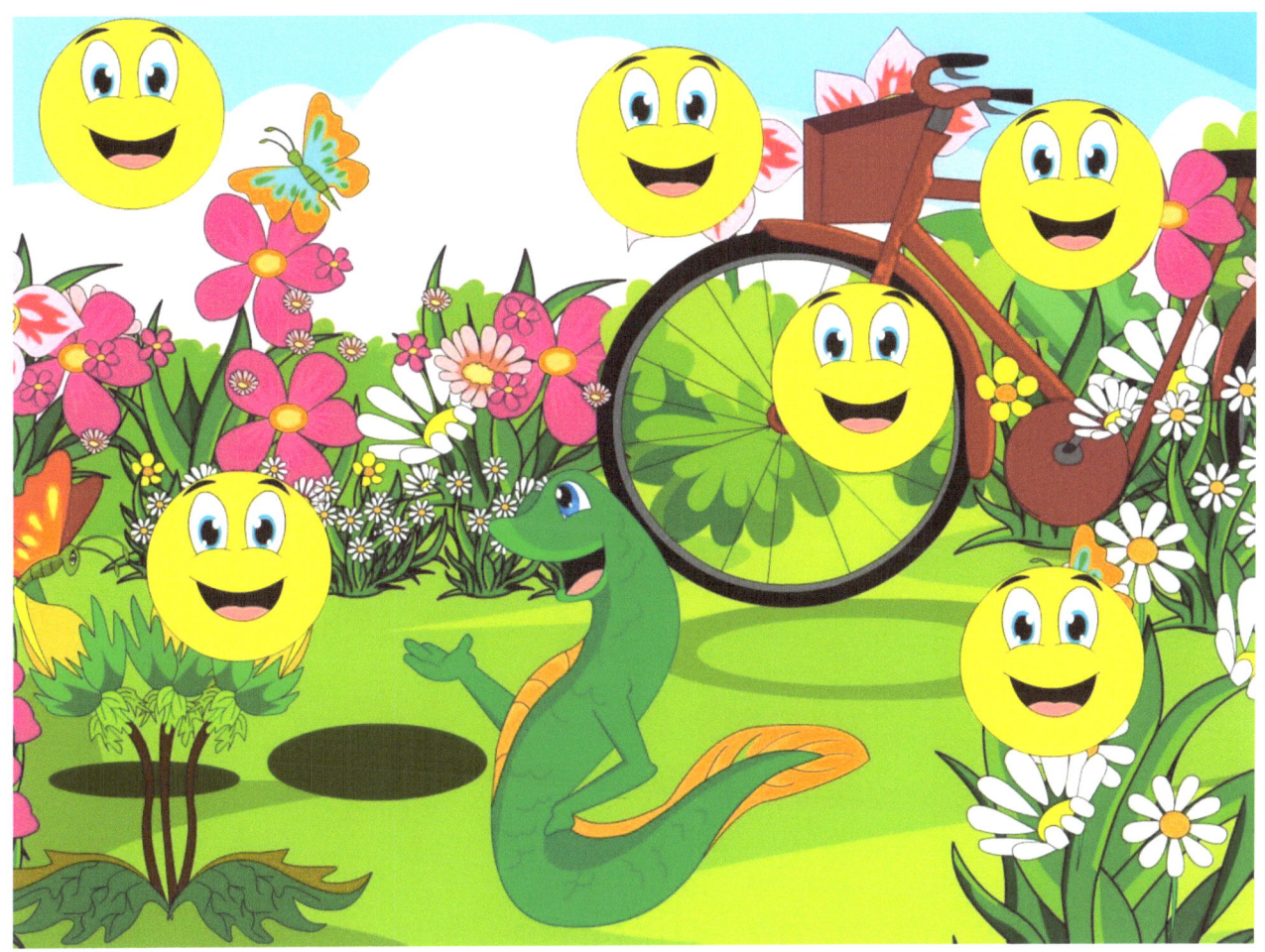

Emily nodded as she calmly mused

"PMA stands for Positive Mental Attitude

A big part of health as you will find

Is not just your body but that of your mind."

"Firstly Oscar, you need to believe in your plan

Believe in yourself and believe that you can

You may not be able to do it quite yet,

But with plenty of practice the better you get"

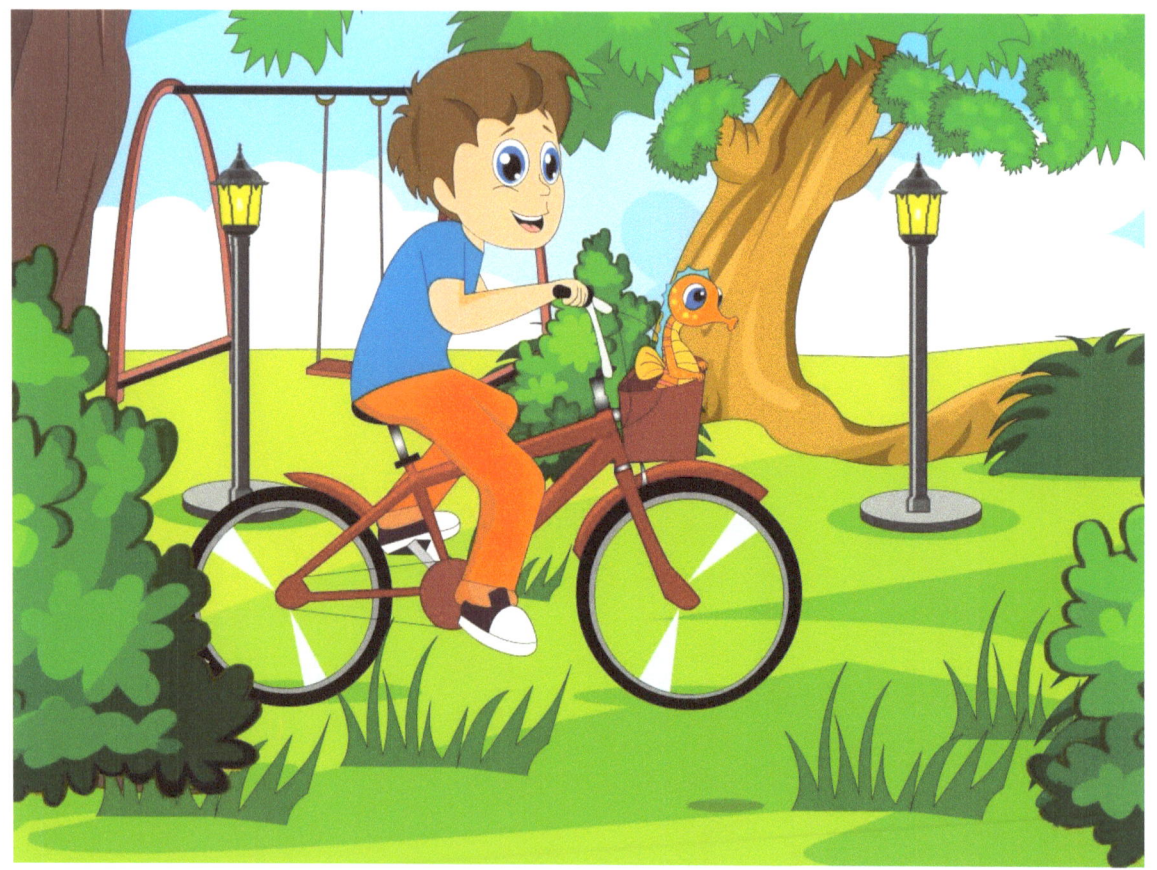

"You take a deep breath, close your eyes and then

Open them, pick up your bike and start again.

Loose that frown and show us your smile

Practice and practice, it does take a while."

Oscar Stood up, stretched and started to move

But he was not there yet, he was not in the groove.

So Jessie Jellyfish decided to help in her way,

"What bothers you Oscar on this bright sunny day?"

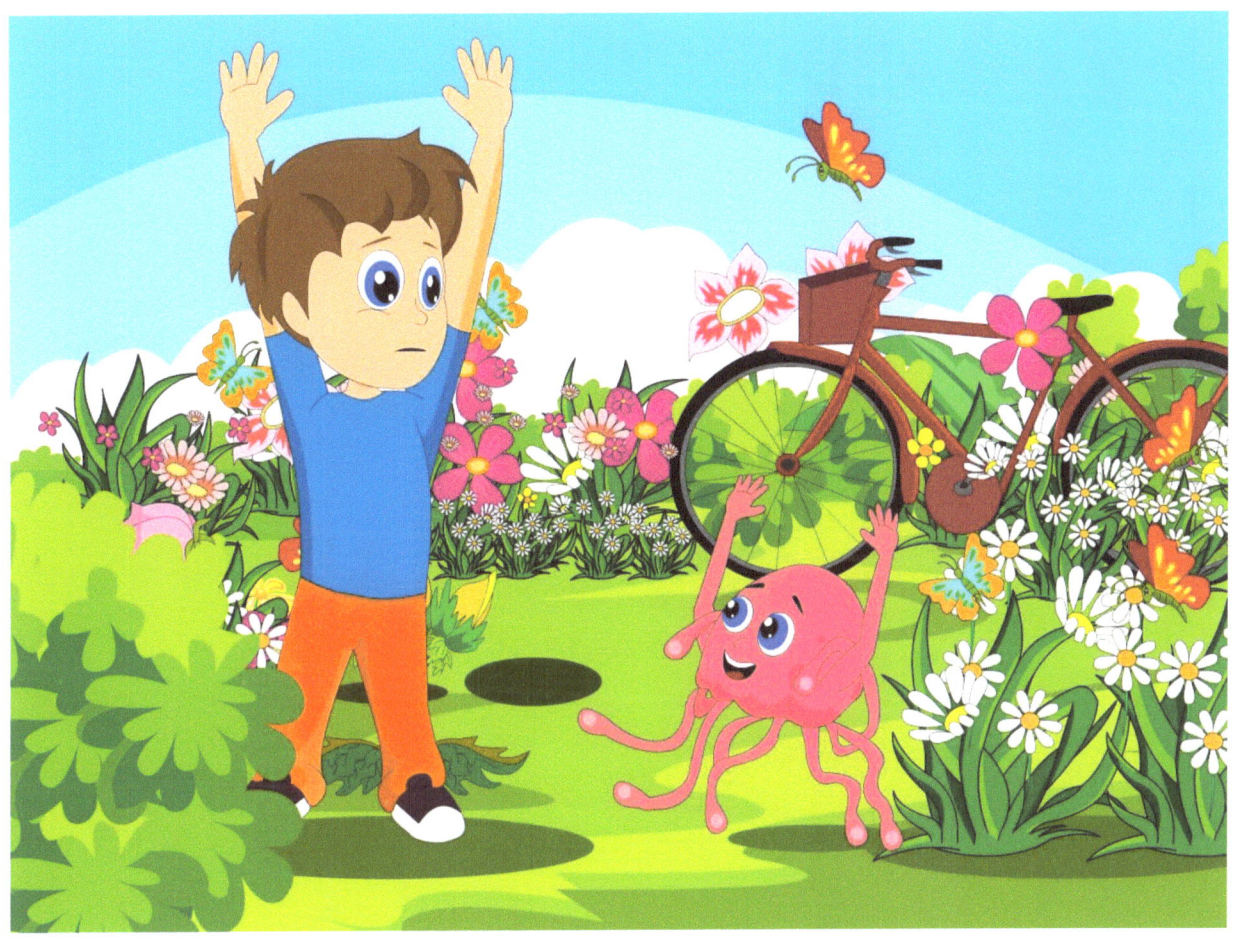

"It's my friends" said Oscar,

Tommy and Oliver

They tell me I'm silly and can't ride

It's true, they are right. I want to hide."

Jessie, put her arm on Oscar's shoulder

It was tensed up so hard and tight as a boulder.

"Oscar," Said Jessie, "you listen to me

You can be, do and have whatever you want you see."

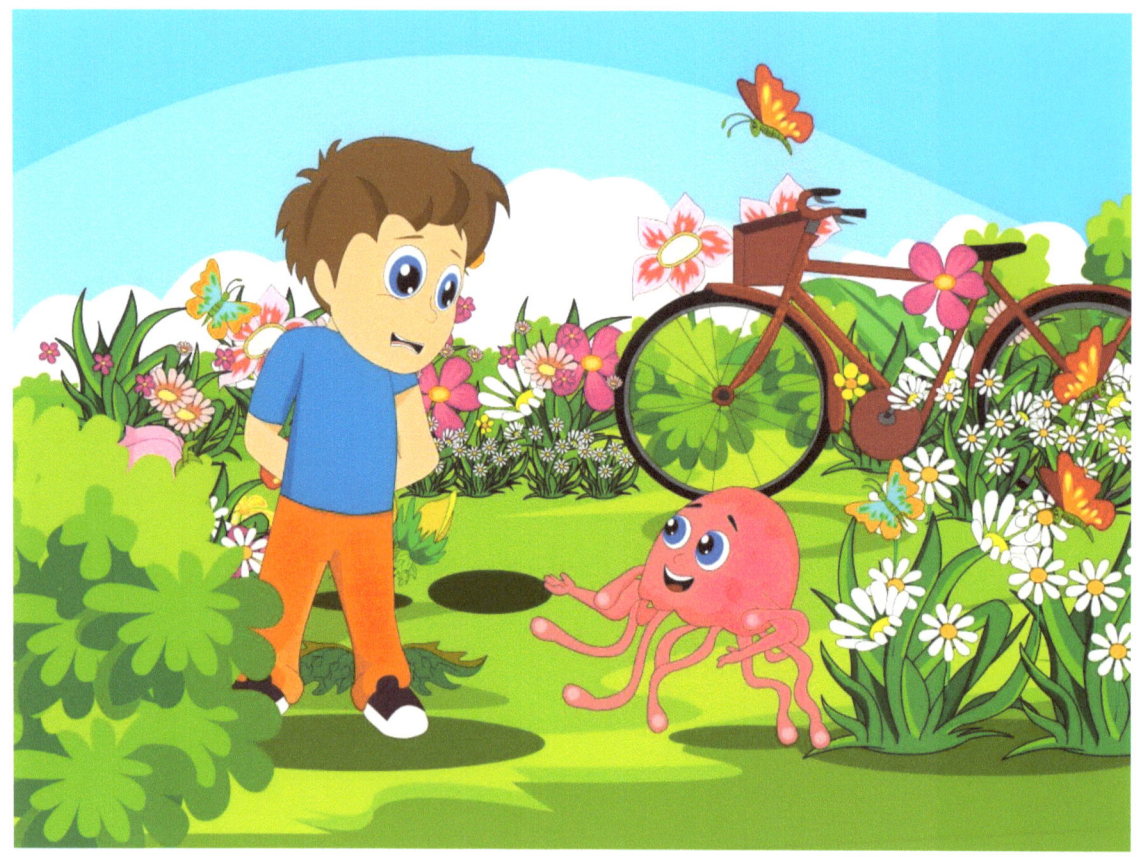

"It can take lots of time and effort and strain,

But on you must go again and again.

Ignore the ones, who only have bad things to say,

They won't help you on your way.

"They will make you sad, lonely and miserable

And that's what we call negative people.

Seek out those that are happy for you

Positive people give love and support, it's true."

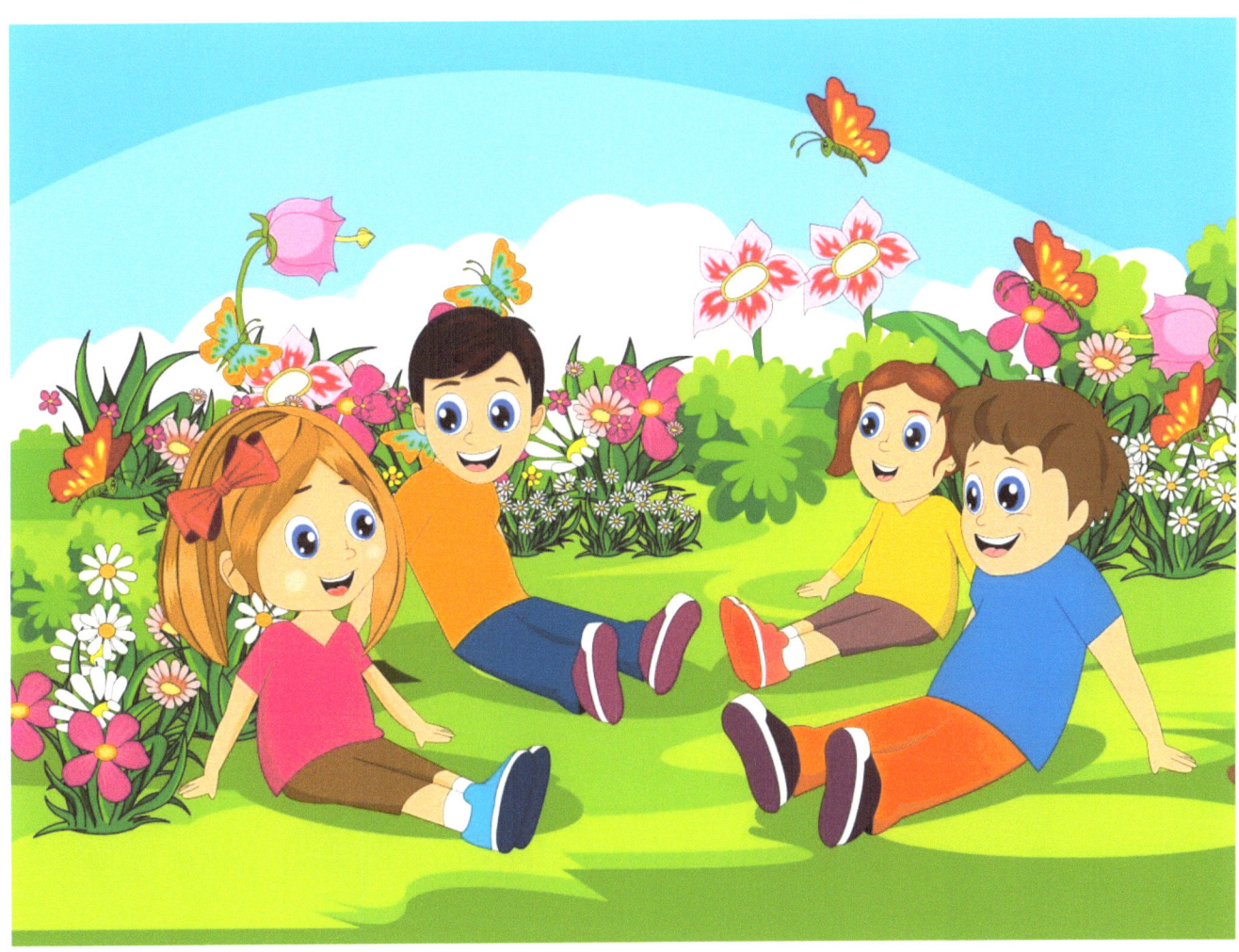

"That's right, Oscar." Sidney Starfish called out

"And now that you have lost that pout.

I want to close your eyes

We are going to reflect and visualise."

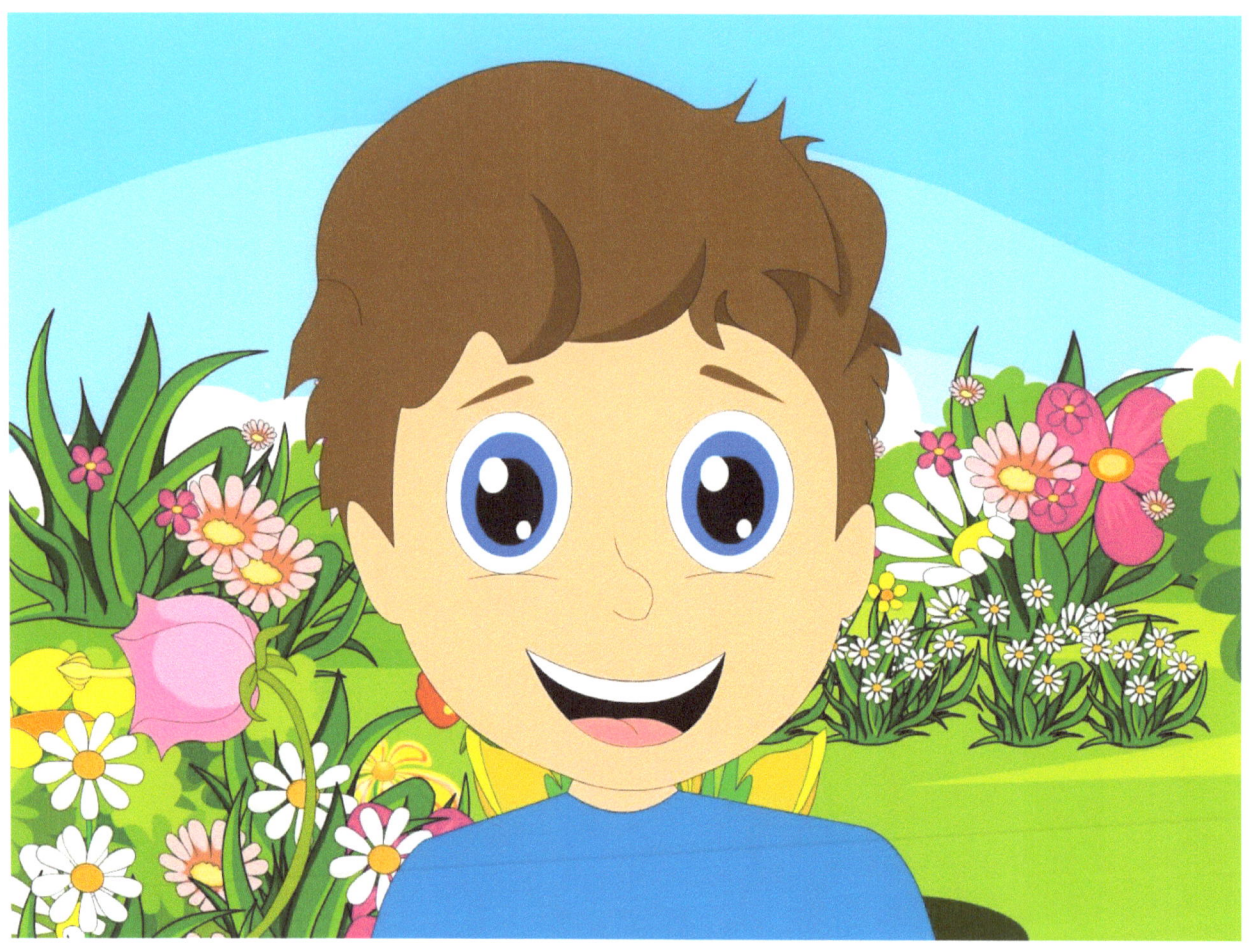

"See yourself riding along on your bike

Riding round fast down by the lake

The air is fresh and the sun's high in the sky

It's beautiful isn't it? And here s why...

"This is your dream, this is what you want

There is no one around who can tell you you can't.

How does this feel to you Oscar?

I bet now you feel happy and stronger.

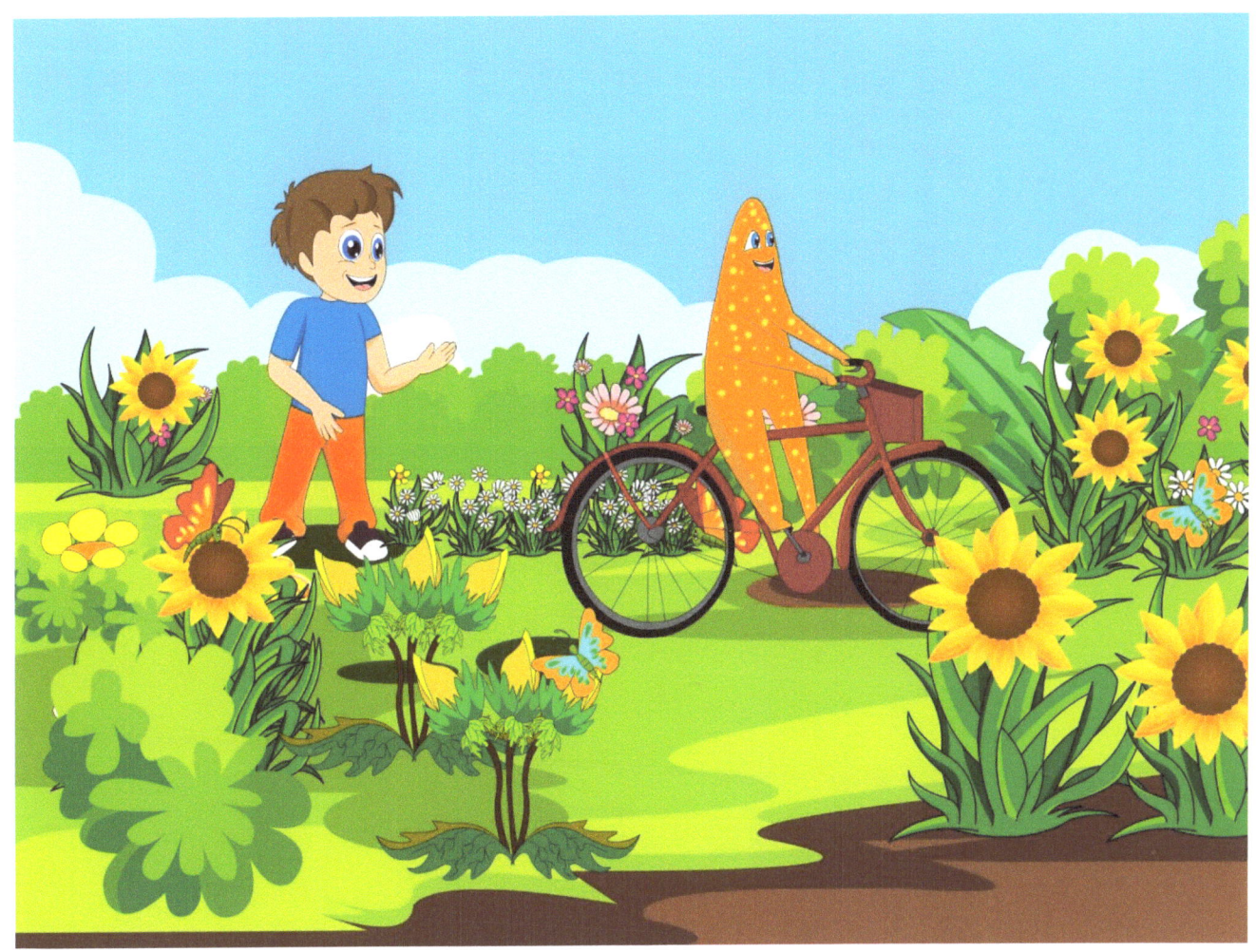

"I do," said Oscar, "but it's so hard

To practice so much I just get bored."

Olga laughed and said, "Oh Oscar you need to stop.

Take regular breaks to keep on top."

"Don't try to do it all at once in a rush.

There is plenty of time Oscar, don't fuss.

Part of the fun is the journey you see,

It's not always smooth, that I agree."

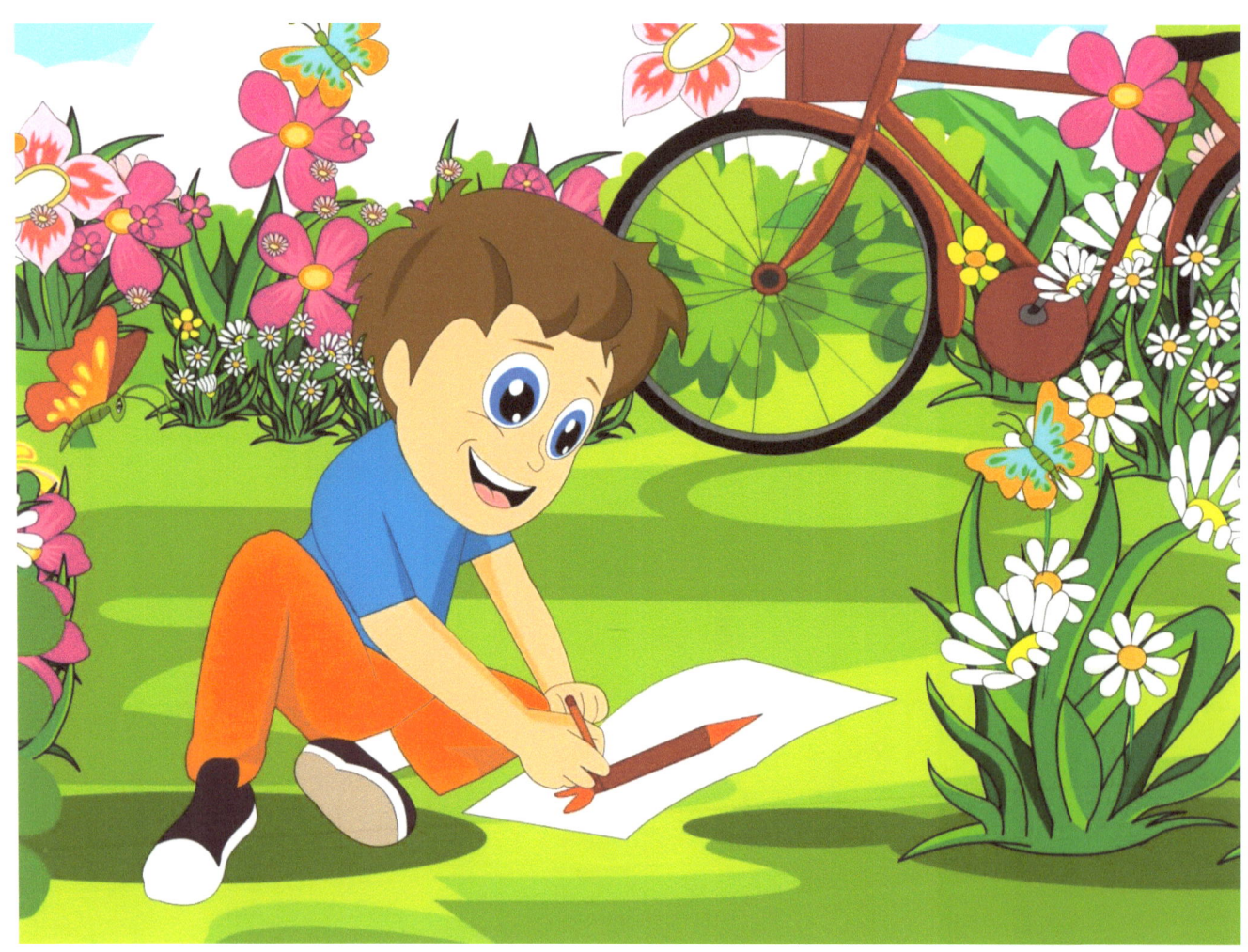

"So go off and do something else for a bit,

Then come back again when you see fit."

"So you see Oscar," Sammy said to his pal,

"We all have times when we must fail,

But then we get up and continue on,

Because we know now where we went wrong."

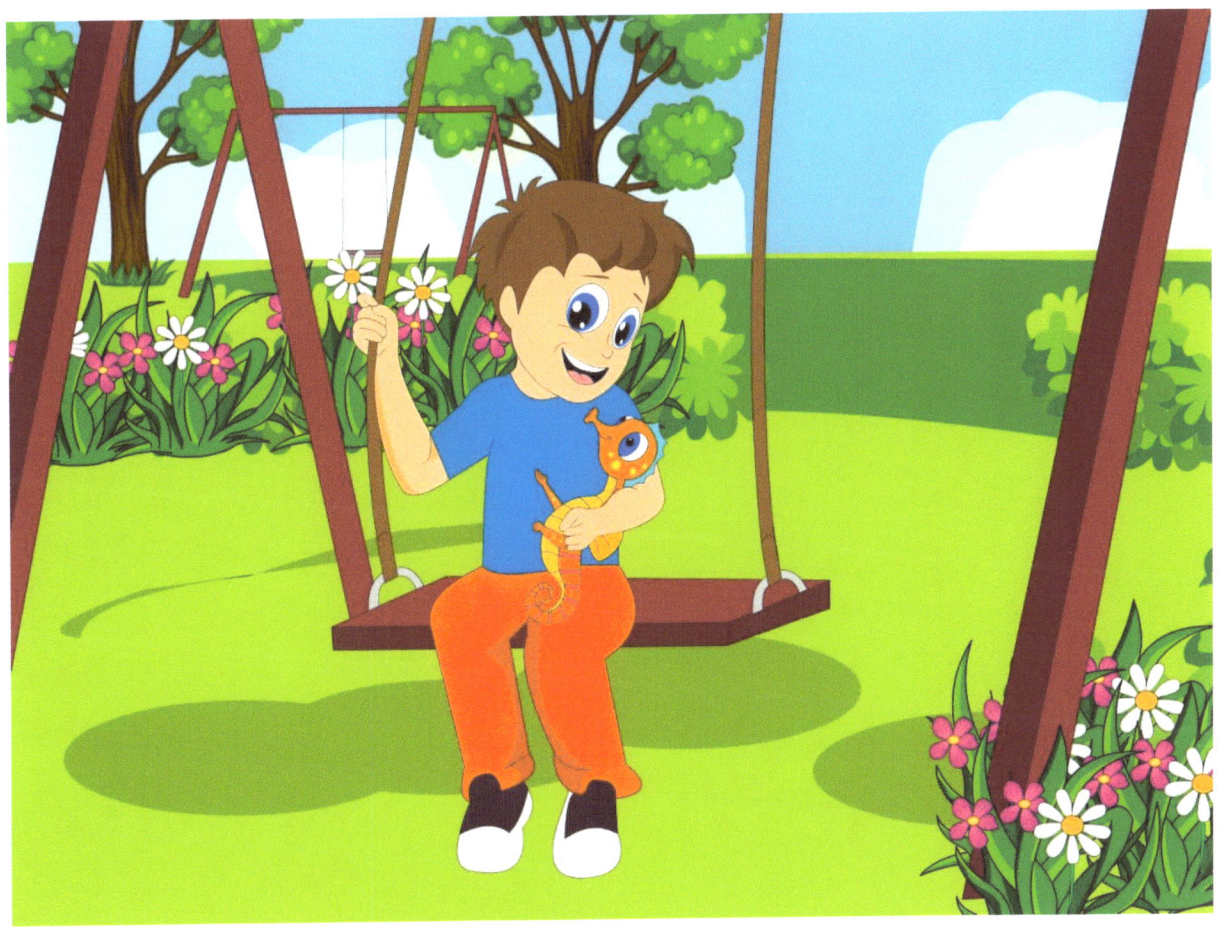

"Making mistakes is part of the plan,

It won't always run smoothly and glam,

But learn from your mistakes you will

And then great success you will feel."

Oscar was now smiling away,

Suddenly everything made sense that day:

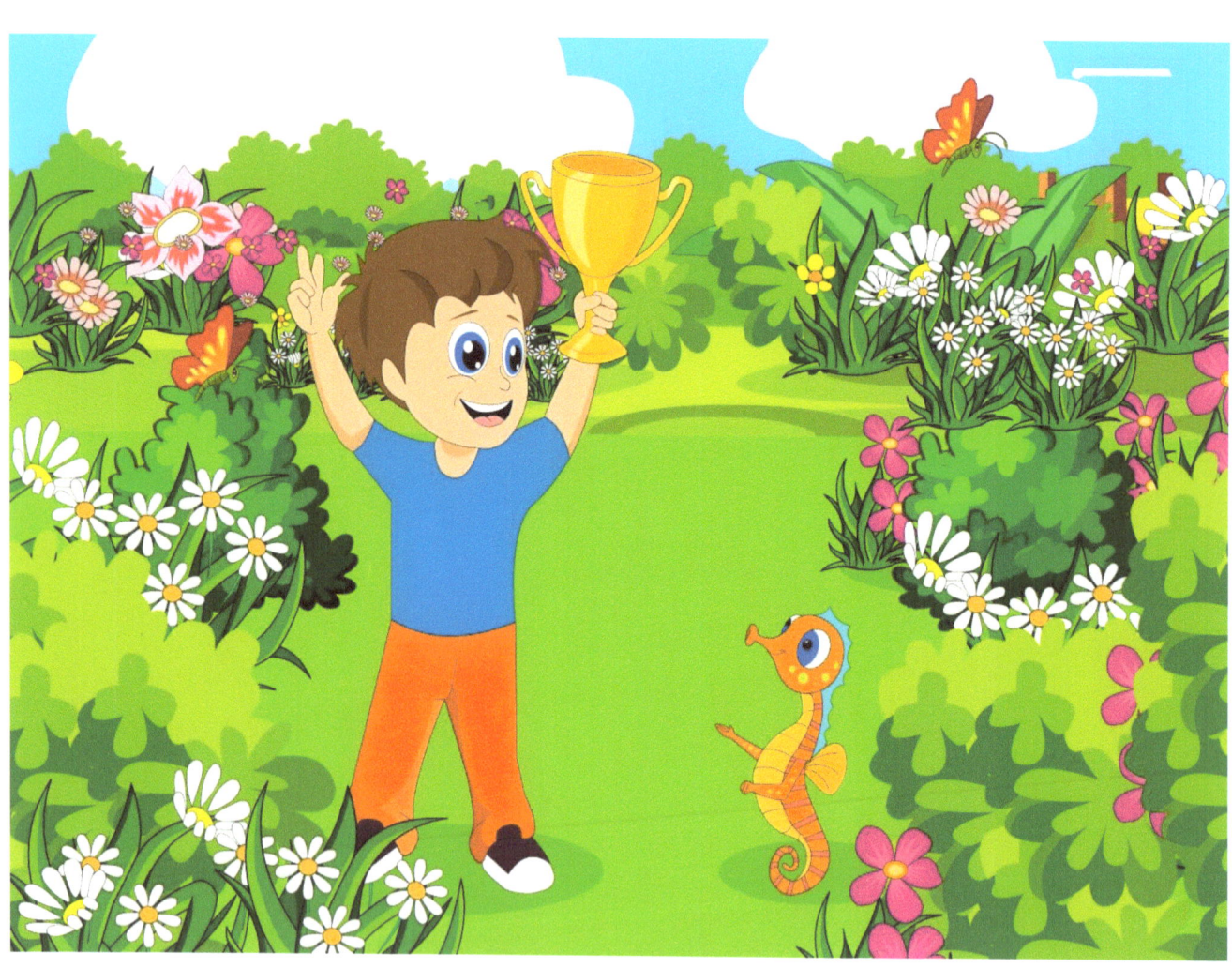

"I may fall off at times, its true;

It's the same with every new thing that we do.

There are many things that are both good and bad,

But we go through them all, and it sounds mad,

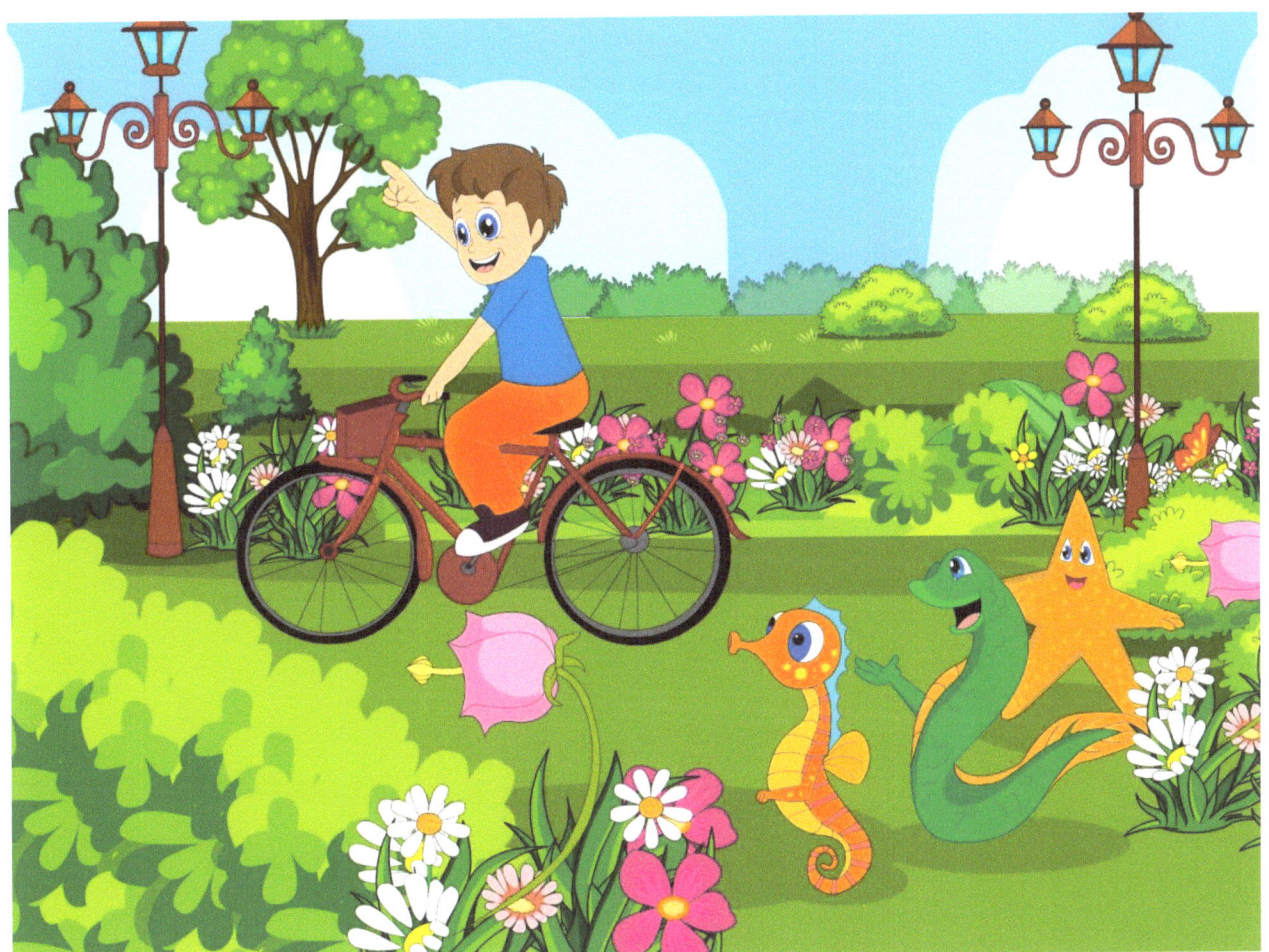

"This is what shapes us and makes us grow.

We can do anything, we just have to know.

PMA is what is important for me

To be the best me that I can be!"

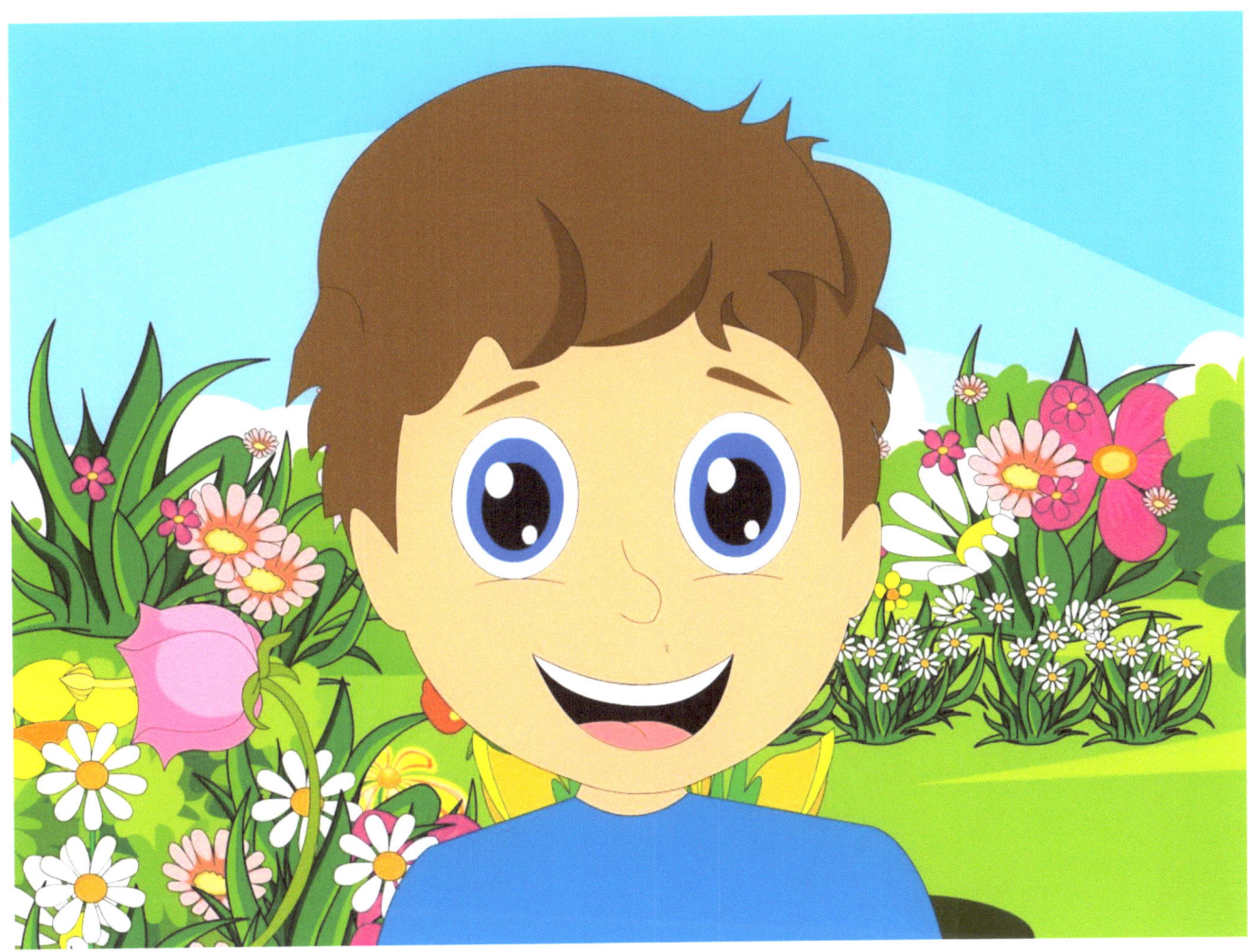

About the Author

Jo Groenhart first developed Oscar Ocean in 2010. Jo had been working at a thriving wellness centre and noticed that many children didn't realise the importance of healthy habits such as sleep, stretching and nutrition and the role these play in leading a healthy lifestyle. She noticed on observing infants that they naturally stretch all the time, it's *in their programming*, however as we grow older we lose this good habit. As education is vital in the early years, it makes sense to encourage good habits and educate our children further.

Jo currently lives in Cambridgeshire with her husband Ed, two sons, Isaac and Oakley, and dog, Izzy. Managing their busy family wellness centre and seeing her own client base has given her an ability to help families create their own wellness lifestyle.

Oscar Ocean and his friend's journey through different adventures in each of the books, exploring the importance of the 7 Habits of Health.

Follow the progress of the rest of Oscar's journey at www.facebook.com/jo.groenhart

JOIN OSCAR AND SAMMY IN THEIR NEXT ADVENTURE, OSCAR OCEAN AND THE BIG SUNSHINE

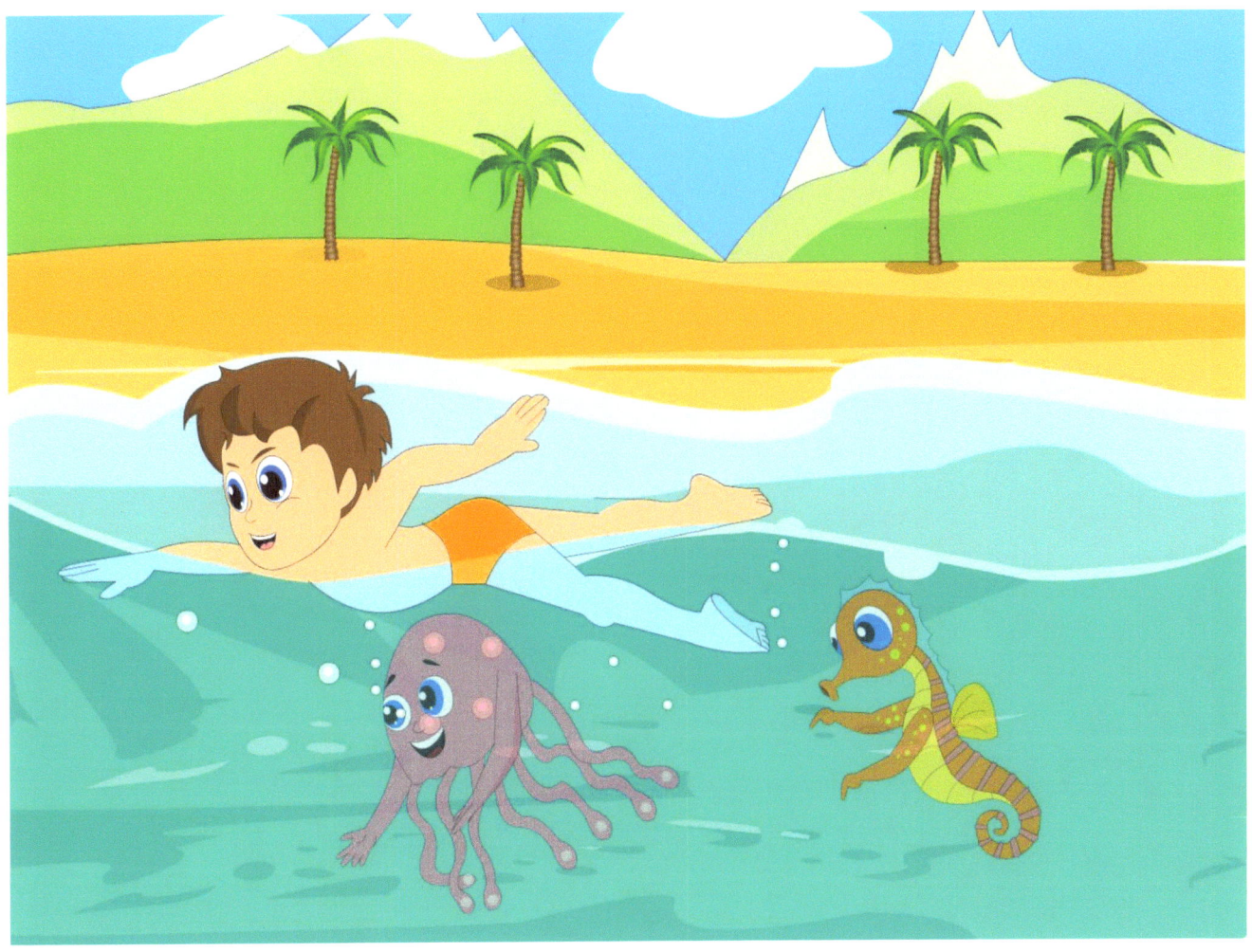

AVAILABLE OCTOBER 2016